THE REDEFINED YOU

A Weight Loss Guide To Help You
Create A Brand New You In Order To
Enjoy A Whole New Life

Dr. Taketa Williams

The Redefined You

ISBN 978-0-98256-893-4
Copyright © 2011 By Exousia Book Publishing

Published By Exousia Book Publishing
Phone: 1-888-424-9673
Website: www.exousiabookpublishing.com or
www.taketawilliamsministries.org

Scripture quotations are used primarily from the King James Version of the Bible.

Scripture quotations marked (AMP) are taken from the Amplified Bible, Copyright © 1954, 1958, 1962, 1964, 1965, 1987 by The Lockman Foundation.

Important Message

Prior to beginning any weight loss process, consult with your physician or health care practitioner to obtain their recommendation and approval.

Table of Contents

Introduction

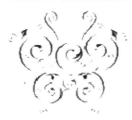

There comes a point and time in life where we get incredibly tired of talking about what we are going to do and finally we make a decision to do what we desire to get done. For at least 5 years straight, I talked about losing weight, tried various weight loss plans, attempted many yo-yo diets, started and stopped exercise regiments and never accomplished any of my weight loss goals. I had so many broken commitments regarding losing weight that I stopped believing myself concerning this matter. I decided that if I wanted others to continue believing in me, then I must first believe in myself, my ability, my potential, and most of all the words that I speak out of my mouth. If I said that I would lose weight and become physically whole, then I had to believe in my own words in order to achieve my objectives and see my words come to pass.

One day I was thinking, planning and preparing for some things that I desired to take place and accomplish in the year ahead of me. All of a sudden, I was interrupted by a spontaneous vision that had speedily popped up on the screen of my mind. I clearly saw the futuristic, glorious, changed me flash before my eyes. I was both overwhelmed and excited about what was mentally and vividly displayed. With a loud voice, I uttered to myself, *"WOW, you look so much better in your future."* This was a Redefining Moment for me and from that time forward I had a true revelation of what I looked like in my future. The new destined me looked to fabulous to forfeit. At that instance an unusual strength came upon me and I could hear a chain break. Immediately, the stronghold that was on my mind regarding the achievement of fitness, weight loss and good health shattered off my paradigm. Instaneously, I felt liberty and a remarkable freedom from the spirit of obesity. I had been set free and was confident that as I made some immediate changes that I would see the results of my deliverance and walk in my breakthrough. I was finally free to become the new me!

I refused to ever be bound again so on April 11, 2011 I launched my own weight loss challenge. I called it the, "Dr. Taketa Williams Redefined Campaign." This time was THE TIME for me. There was something different about my commitment than any other moment before. The feeling I had was supernatural. I knew I was not operating on mere desire, but I sensed a release into my destiny. In order to embark upon destiny, it requires an anointing – a supernatural ability to do what could not ordinary be done before. In my gut, I felt like what I was getting ready to do was already done and all I had to do was walk in it. The way was made and the pathway was prepared. As my spiritual brother and friend, Bishop Greg Davis, says I just had to GOGETIT! This was a Redefining Moment in my life and I was determined not to miss it. My life was about to be changed forever.

On this campaign, I was determined not to fail therefore I established an accountability system and shared my plans with a team of people that would inspire me to follow through with my obligation to become redefined. When I publicly stated my aspiration to become physically fit and lose weight, it forced me to do exactly what I said I would do. As a sought after preacher and public figure, I knew many watched me, looked up to me and believed my words. If I didn't do what I declared, then I would have lost credibility. I refused to allow that to happen, therefore I remained true to my word.

You must have a system of accountability in place that will help hold you responsible for becoming the new you that you said you would be. Tell your family, your friends, your coworkers and other supporters what your plans are and give them permission to hold you accountable. I openly communicated what my goals were. I said that I would lose at least 60 pounds in four months and that I would exercise on a faithful and consistent basis. I recreated my new eating ethics and shared with others exactly what I ate. Refer to the workbook for a list of menu choices and food options that will assist you with weight loss. In addition, I would share my results as the weight came off.

Along the way I practiced celebrating my accomplishments. Applaud your successes even if they seem small. In any given week if you only lose a 1/2 of a pound, celebrate that. Don't become discouraged even if your achievements seem very minor and minute. Every little bit counts and ultimately becomes much when you remain persistent. Publicize your results and share them with those that are happy for you. You will acquire some critics and haters along the way, but stay focused. Some people are negative by nature and it's simply not in them to say anything positive and complimentary. Just keep doing you and, in everything, endeavor to be thankful regarding your progress. Keep an optimistic mindset and don't allow anyone or anything to get you off track. Remember, you are working on something and you have a goal that you must reach. Whatever you desire to accomplish is in your reach but you must keep stretching forward no matter what with intense passion and steadfast determination.

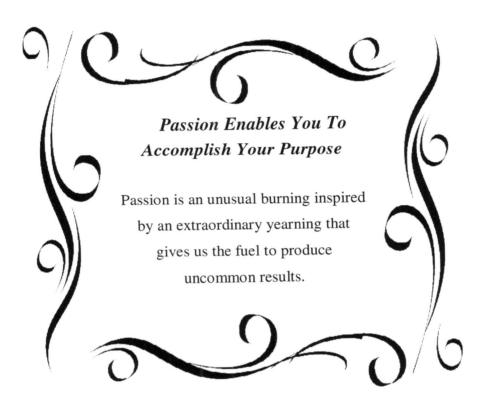

Passion Enables You To Accomplish Your Purpose

Passion is an unusual burning inspired
by an extraordinary yearning that
gives us the fuel to produce
uncommon results.

Chapter One

Redefine You Today!

Bring new meaning to your life by redefining you. You have the opportunity to create your own definition of who you are and what you represent. Don't allow life's circumstances or the opinions of other people to define you. Make a bold statement and tell the world who you are instead of waiting on someone else to affirm what you were born to be. You can only be THE YOU that you know you to be. If you don't know who you are then you can't fully be. Your existence becomes obsolete and your purpose will remain unknown. There is a you that is waiting to be created and you have the power to do it by redefining yourself today.

Redefining your life begins with getting a revelation of who you are in your future. Life is so much more satisfying and rewarding when your identity matches your destiny or, more specifically, when who you are now is exactly what you were always meant to be later. It is important that you begin to look like today who you were created to be tomorrow. Your future is now and you must begin to resemble the futuristic you immediately.

How much do you weigh in your future? What size do you wear one year from now? What's the condition of your health in 6 months? These are questions you must ask yourself in order to determine who you are getting ready to become. When you obtain a revelation of the new you, write it out and have an artist sketch exactly what you saw. Frame the picture of who you will be so that you can use it as a guide to become it. It is vitally necessary that you write your vision and make it plain. When you read it then you will be empowered to run with it. Remember, without a vision you will perish and never become who you were born to be.

What is it to redefine oneself?

Primarily, to redefine is to define again. This meaning implies that you once had meaning but somewhere along the way you lost it and are in need of acquiring it again. Often times, we lose definition through lack of recognition. Along the way, we fail to recognize who we are because we get swallowed up by the opinions of others that tell us who we aren't. *When you know emphatically who you are, you don't allow anyone to tell you who you aren't.* The greatest voice in your life should be God and you. You should be confident in both who He says you are and who you say you are. There is an unusual confidence that is unshakable that emanates from a person that has been redefined and rebirthed in the earth. People's opinions of you no longer dictate to you your essence or discourage you from enjoying your existence. You have resolved within yourself who you are and have become exactly what you thought. Indeed, you are exactly what you think. You have a second chance to re-exist and begin to live again. If you can define it, think it, and articulate it, then you will become it. Pronunciation coupled with determination causes an astonishing realization. What you say and what you think will go from being a dream into a wonderful reality.

Write down on paper who you are then formulate your own definition. Declare out of your mouth and decree it on the tablets of your heart. If you decree a thing, it will be established. When you write it or decree it, it becomes a law and when you say it or declare it becomes life. There's death and life in the power of your tongue. Say who you are so you can live to be who you desire to be.

Example definition:

I am a 140 pound bold, beautiful, knock em' dead gorgeous, powerful, wealthy and elite lady. I am healthy and the fruit of my body is blessed. I am physically, mentally, emotionally, sexually and spiritually, economically and financially fit. I live a holistic prosperous life. I am attractive and I attract only what I am. I am blessed therefore I attract only blessed people and blessed things to my life.

Write your name and the meaning of who you are.
Create your own definition of you here:

Your Name

_____

Your Definition of the New You

_____

_____

_____

Secondly, to redefine is to reformulate. When you reformulate a thing it requires that you reexamine or reevaluate especially with the mindset to change or update. Systems run better and much faster when they are updated and upgraded. Change is a great part of being upgraded. Upgrading consists of purging out old clutter from the system that slowed down its function and adding new tools and software that will enhance its performance. Your body is a system and must be reformulated and upgraded if you want it to operate at its full potential. Reformulating includes devising and developing a method or formula to aid in the updating process. When formulating your system, determine what works best for your body. A low-fat, low carb, low calorie formula worked best for me. Have your doctor, dietician or nutritionist help you determine what is most effective for you and your body type.

In order to become redefined, you must endure your process of change. Without making the necessary changes in your life and habits, the redefining process can never begin. Reexamine where you are and reevaluate what is required to get to where you need to go. I assure you that you will make it and arrive at your destination. You must be honest with yourself and have a good self-talk about everything that you don't like about you so that you can become more likeable by transforming your dislikes into great likes. If you don't like your current weight, your outward appearance or your physical features, you have the power to change them. Change is not always easy however it is doable. YOU CAN DO IT. It can be quite laborious, but hard work will pay off and you will achieve the results you want if you stick with your plan.

Thirdly, to redefine is to state or set forth the meaning of. Life is more meaningful when your existence has meaning. It's knowing who you are and being fulfilled with that person that provides more definition to living. When you mean something then life means something. You must state exactly who you are and then who you are will be set forth and manifest. Don't be ashamed or intimidated to declare your meaning. The more you say it, the more you will see it.

Declare daily, I am 50 pounds lighter. I am free from all sickness and diseases. I am in perfect health. I am physically fit. I am satisfied with long life. I am free from the power of low self-esteem. I possess great confidence. I am a dazzling star and I shine best at night. Say it and people will see it on you and in you.

There comes a time in your life where you simply get sick and tired of where you are and you become desperate for change to take place. During this moment, you make a conscious internal decision to do something extremely different to attain different results. We all know that it is insanity to continue to do the same thing over and over again expecting a different outcome. I was simply fed up with my weight and my size. I had to be honest with me and tell myself, *"You are beautiful, anointed and very powerful, but you're FAT."* As an adult, I always knew I was gorgeous but bodacious − simply big and beautiful. I admired the beauty but I did not prefer the big. I conformed to the way I was and finally realized it was a hindrance to who I was to become. That wasn't cool anymore to me. Rather or not it was with others didn't matter; it simply wasn't acceptable to me. I no longer wanted to be like I was, fat, obese and overweight.

As a result of obesity, my health began to suffer tremendously. I said to myself it's a shame that you preach the word, move in power, cast out devils and heal the sick, but you're unhealthy yourself. I began to feel like a castaway and a reproach. How could I command sugar diabetes to leave somebody else when it had a hold on me? The condition of my health began to offend my anointing. My spirit became agitated with my flesh. My flesh had become an enemy to my spirit and started to sap-suck the power that I possessed within. This disease had set in and would wear me out physically. Many days I would have to borrow spiritual power to give me the physical strength to preach the word and minister to God's people because my sugar levels had drained me tremendously. *I would travel the world, arrive to the best hotels, and engage many pulpits with abnormal blood sugar levels of 250-300. (See facts and data about diabetes on pages 20-23.)* At once, it registered in my mind popping diabetes pills and prophesying weren't a good mix. Something had to give and there were some things that I had to give up.

I would eat all the wrong foods. My norm on various occasions was like a Thanksgiving feast on a regular Friday night. My abundant spread was endowed with fried chicken, smothered pork chops with gravy, oxtails over white rice, greens with ham hock, macaroni and cheese, sweet potatoes loaded with sugar and syrup, cakes, pies and whatever else I wanted accompanied by a diet soda. The diet soda had a way of tricking my brain and convincing me that what I was taking in my body wasn't so bad. In fact, it was beyond bad, it was horrible and absolutely disgusting. I decided to change and realized that I was an agent of change in the earth. I concluded with knowing that if I had helped others to change then surely I could change myself.

Finally, I meant what I said and I said what I meant then new meaning to life and the new me was set forth. I said it, I meant it, and I birthed it – the brand new me.

The weight fell off expediently and within 4 ½ months I had lost 70! Both me and life were redefined and I fell in love again with the born again me!

To Redefine Is

To Define Again

To Reformulate

To State or Set Forth the Meaning of

Facts about Obesity and Diabetes

About one-third of U.S. adults (33.8%) are obese. Approximately 17% (or 12.5 million) of children and adolescents aged 2—19 years are obese.

Data from the National Health and Examination Survey (NHANES)

Your Culture Can Aid In Obesity

During the past 20 years, there has been a dramatic increase in obesity in the United States and rates remain high. In 2010, no state had a prevalence of obesity less than 20%. Thirty-six states had a prevalence of 25% or more; 12 of these states (Alabama, Arkansas, Kentucky, Louisiana, Michigan, Mississippi, Missouri, Oklahoma, South Carolina, Tennessee, Texas, and West Virginia) had a prevalence of 30% or more.

What is Obesity?

Obesity Word Origin & History

1610s, from Fr. obésité, from L. obesitas "fatness, corpulence," from obesus "that has eaten itself fat," pp. of obdere "to eat all over, devour," from ob "over" + edere "eat". *When we operate in obesity, we resemble like Satan. He is a devourer. According to the Word of the Lord, God is rebukes devourers for His name sake.*

From Online Etymology Dictionary, © 2010 Douglas Harper

According to the World English Dictionary obesity is a condition that is characterized by excessive accumulation and storage of fat in the body and that in an adult is typically indicated by a body mass index (BMI) of 30 or greater.

BMI Ranges:	
Underweight	< 20
Ideal	20-25
Overweight	25-30
Obese	> 30

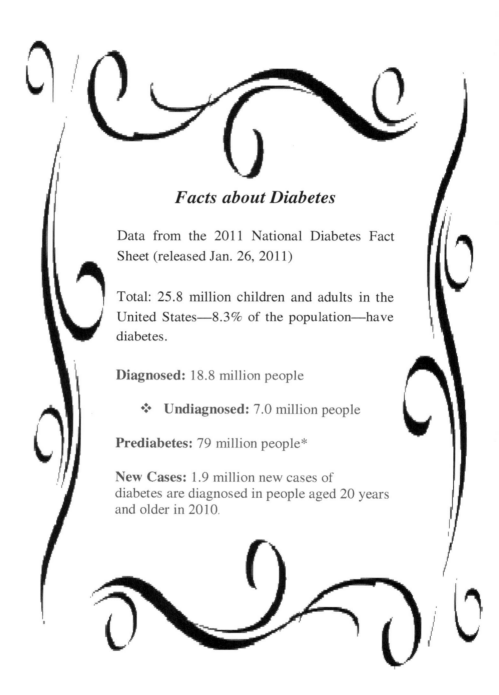

Facts about Diabetes

Data from the 2011 National Diabetes Fact Sheet (released Jan. 26, 2011)

Total: 25.8 million children and adults in the United States—8.3% of the population—have diabetes.

Diagnosed: 18.8 million people

❖ **Undiagnosed:** 7.0 million people

Prediabetes: 79 million people*

New Cases: 1.9 million new cases of diabetes are diagnosed in people aged 20 years and older in 2010.

Race and ethnic differences in prevalence of diagnosed diabetes

After adjusting for population age differences, 2007-2009 national survey data for people diagnosed with diabetes, aged 20 years or older include the following prevalence by race/ethnicity:

- 7.1% of non-Hispanic whites
- 8.4% of Asian Americans
- 12.6% of non-Hispanic blacks
- 11.8% of Hispanics

Among Hispanics rates were:

- 7.6% for Cubans
- 13.3% for Mexican Americans
- 13.8% for Puerto Ricans.

Morbidity and Mortality

- In 2007, diabetes was listed as the underlying cause on 71,382 death certificates and was listed as a contributing factor on an additional 160,022 death certificates. This means that diabetes contributed to a total of 231,404 deaths.

Dangers and Complications of Diabetes

Heart disease and stroke

- In 2004, heart disease was noted on 68% of diabetes-related death certificates among people aged 65 years or older.
- In 2004, stroke was noted on 16% of diabetes-related death certificates among people aged 65 years or older.
- Adults with diabetes have heart disease death rates about 2 to 4 times higher than adults without diabetes.
- The risk for stroke is 2 to 4 times higher among people with diabetes.

High blood pressure

- In 2005-2008, of adults aged 20 years or older with self-reported diabetes, 67% had blood pressure greater than or equal to 140/90 mmHg or used prescription medications for hypertension.

Blindness

- Diabetes is the leading cause of new cases of blindness among adults aged 20–74 years.
- In 2005-2008, 4.2 million (28.5%) people with diabetes aged 40 years or older had diabetic

retinopathy, and of these, almost 0.7 million (4.4% of those with diabetes) had advanced diabetic retinopathy that could lead to severe vision loss.

Dangers and Complications of Diabetes Continued

Kidney disease

- Diabetes is the leading cause of kidney failure, accounting for 44% of new cases in 2008.
- In 2008, 48,374 people with diabetes began treatment for end-stage kidney disease in the United States.
- In 2008, a total of 202,290 people with end-stage kidney disease due to diabetes were living on chronic dialysis or with a kidney transplant in the United States.

Nervous system disease (Neuropathy)

- About 60% to 70% of people with diabetes have mild to severe forms of nervous system damage.

Amputation

- More than 60% of non-traumatic lower-limb amputations occur in people with diabetes.
- In 2006, about 65,700 non-traumatic lower-limb amputations were performed in people with diabetes.

Chapter Two

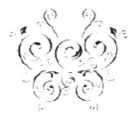

Where To Begin?

First, make a decision to change now in order to get the results you want later. You are one decision away from a greater and much more incredible you. Let's not focus on the amount of weight you have to lose, instead concentrate on the new life you will gain. If you focus on losing, then you will acquire a losing attitude and end up forfeiting your weight loss success. Think about all the things that you will gain. During my process, so much was added to my life. My emotional life, mental life, sexual life, physical life and recreational life all were enhanced greatly. I finally felt comfortable in the skin I was in. I no longer looked and felt like a loaded, stuffed baked potato running over with extra butter and sour cream. I was transformed into a wonderful chef salad that I uniquely created. I became full of flavor, pizzazz and an array of color – low fat and full of nutrients! I simply gained a new found abundant, blessed, and blissful life. You simply have to give up something in order to get something greater. Trust me. Giving up the wrong things and embracing the right choices will bring about mind blowing results that will make you step back, look in the mirror and say, WOW, I can't believe it's not butter!

Make the decision to become a part of a winning team and a victorious you. When you make a decision, great things begin to happen. One great man once said, "When you make a decision, the universe conspires to make it happen." Everything in you and around you begins to synergistically work together to help make happen what you desire to be so. If you decide it, believe it and work hard at it, then you can have it. You can have whatever you say. Keep saying it and you have no choice but to see it. Confess daily that you are fit, you are fat-free, you are fierce, you are super fine, full of passion and on fire, hot and the smoking whip! When you show up, people should smell smoke! The new you will cause heads to turn, eyes to gaze and people will be utterly amazed by the Redefined, Brand New you!

After making your decision to redefine you, don't renege on your commitment. Stick to it no matter what. There will be many things that will rise up against you in attempt to distract you and get you off track. You must be determined to stay your course. If you give into the distractions, it will cause a great delay in achieving the results that you want. Your body can only become what you create it to be through diligence and consistency. When I was out of shape and overweight, I diligently over ate and consistently indulged foods that were not healthy to my body. Stick to your process! It will be worth your while and your results will be phenomenal.

Next, launch your Personal Redefined Campaign. During your campaign, determine what you want to accomplish by the conclusion of your process. Keep in mind, that in order to avoid becoming discouraged and disappointed about your weight loss endeavor, it is important that you are realistic about what you want to accomplish. If you really want to SMAC defeat and gain the victory during your campaign, then your goals should be **S**pecific, **M**easurable, **A**ttainable and **C**onsistent.

Now let's establish your goals by answering these questions.

How much do you currently weight? _____

How long have you been dissatisfied with your present weight? _____

How much weight do you desire to lose? _____

What is your present clothes size? _____

What size clothing do you desire to wear? _____

What is the time frame in which you want   to lose your excess weight? _____

What are the target areas on your body that you would like to focus on improving? _____

What health issues do you have that are caused and/or agitated because of poor eating habits? _____

_____

_____

_____

Note: Many medical conditions can be resolved simply through a proper diet and consistent exercise. It is important and necessary that you speak with your physician and obtain their consent before beginning any weight loss or diet and exercise program.

Chapter Three

Let's Get Started

Take a picture of what you look like now. This will motivate you greatly. If you don't like how you look, you have the power to change it! You deserve to be upgraded and should be pleased and proud of your appearance.

*Place Your Pre Redefined Campaign Picture Here
and Get Ready To Create A New You!*

Size Yourself Up!

*

Beginning Weight _____

Waist _____ Inches

Hip _____ Inches

Thigh _____ Inches

Arm _____ Inches

Neck _____ Inches

Identify everything about your appearance that you don't like and that you are determined to change.

_____ Fat Stomach   _____ Huge Thighs

_____ Love Handles and Rolls   _____ Large Arms

_____ Double Chin   _____ Saggy Skin

_____Oversized Neck   _____ Enlarged
                                            Chest

If you have more dislikes, please list below.

_____   _____

_____   _____

_____   _____

_____   _____

All your dislikes are now your areas of focus. You can never change what you are not willing to confront. If you have a fat stomach, then get ready to confront it. Ignoring it will only make matters worse. You have the potential to gain the victory over your condition through your hard work and persistent endeavor. Don't feel pressured to concentrate on all your target areas all at once. Choose at least 2 areas to work on at a time. If you try to aggressively resolve your issues all at the same time, you will become overwhelmed and eventually quit your process.

During the initial phase of my campaign, I worked my stomach and my arms. Most of my weight was lodged in my stomach area; therefore I tackled my biggest area of resistance first. I was disgusted with the way my stomach looked and refused to continue to wait to do something about it. My stomach was entirely too big and it became very unattractive to me. My husband did not have a problem with it; however I began to abhor it. It was simply time for it to go and whatever I had to do to make it leave is what I was willing to do. I was determined and wasn't stopping because I knew exactly what I did and did not want.

Identifying Your Goals

What is a Goal?

A goal is the result or achievement toward which effort is directed; an aim; your end.

Goals initiate new beginnings and will lead you to your ultimate end. Without realistic goals, you will never cross over the finish line. You will find yourself in a place will you keep starting over, stopping then starting over again. In order to achieve any goal it requires that you forget about the past and apprehend intense focus to look towards your future. Your potential achievement cannot be attained without focus. Your initial decision will get you on track, but focus will keep you on track! Don't get off track because it may cost you the race and sabotage your intended success.

Let's Set Some Goals

Start by setting least 3 Specific, Measurable, Attainable and Consistent goals and stick with them no matter what!

Specific Goal #1:

_____

_____

How do you plan to measure this goal?

_____

_____

Is this goal realistic and truly attainable?

_____

_____

How consistent are you with sticking to doing what it takes to accomplish this goal?

_____

_____

When you reach this goal and then be sure to celebrate yourself and record your accomplishment!

Specific Goal #2:

_____

_____

How do you plan to measure this goal?

_____

_____

Is this goal realistic and truly attainable?

_____

_____

How consistent are you with sticking to doing what it takes to accomplish this goal?

_____

_____

When you reach this goal and then be sure to celebrate yourself and record your accomplishment!

Specific Goal #3:

_____

_____

How do you plan to measure this goal?

_____

_____

Is this goal realistic and truly attainable?

_____

_____

How consistent are you with sticking to doing what it takes to accomplish this goal?

_____

_____

When you reach this goal and then be sure to celebrate yourself and record your accomplishment!

Chapter Four

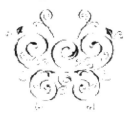

Losing Weight Is Hard Work

If you think that losing excess weight is easy and happens overnight, you are sadly mistaken. It takes time, effort, persistency, focus and lots of energy. The weight did not come upon you overnight so please don't expect it to come off that way. It will take time, however hard work will cut down the time tremendously. I was able to lose 70 pounds in 4 and ½ months which is rare and quite extreme. I changed my diet, exercised at least 6 days per week and drank only water. Alter your diet and caloric intake according to how rapid and how much weight you desire to lose. My plan was quite aggressive because of what I wanted to accomplish.

I cut out all fried foods and eliminated sweets such as cakes, pies, candies and ice cream. Also, I avoided starchy foods like white rice, all potatoes and white breads. Usually if what you eat is white it's not right. Periodically, I would eat a very small portion of brown rice or have a slice of low calorie wheat bread. This would actually trick my body and assure it that I was not starving it. One of my favorite meals that provided me with lots of energy and a suitable amount of fiber was oatmeal. It will not harm you to have a cup of oatmeal daily or several times per week. Oatmeal is low in calories, fat and cholesterol. It is also loaded with fiber and has the right carbohydrates that will provide the body with fuel to burn. If you eat oatmeal, I would definitely recommend that you eat it in the morning for breakfast. This gives your body time to burn off its' carbohydrates.

Losing weight is a formula. In order to lose one pound, you will have to burn at least 3500 calories. With a lower calorie diet and a regular workout schedule, losing a few pounds a week is realistic. I personally did not take in more than 800 calories per day and burned between 500-800 calories per workout. Everyone's needs and ambitions are different. Check with your physician to determine what works best for you.

What it takes to lose a pound?

A pound of body fat equates to approximately 3500 calories. So if you have a calorie deficit of 500 calories (meaning that you burn 500 calories more than you eat each day) you would lose approximately one pound per week: 500 x 7 = 3,500 *(from caloriesperhour.com)*

Weighing In

I would recommend that you weigh yourself twice per week – once at the beginning and once at the end of the week. This will help keep you focused over the weekend which is the time that people are more prone to fall off the weight loss wagon. When weighing in, do it when you wake up prior to putting anything in your body. I have experienced that in the morning is better because you also burn calories while sleeping.

Yes you do burn calories while sleeping!

A 150 pound person can burn around 500 calories during an 8 hour night's sleep. Someone who is 300 pounds could burn just over 1,000 calories. You may not be pumping iron in your sleep, but your body continues to burn energy as your heart keeps pumping and other body systems carry on their work.

Getting your proper rest and adequate sleep is very necessary during your Weight Loss Process.

The number of hours you sleep each night can have an effect on the number of calories you burn. Medical News Today reports that a lack of sleep may alter your metabolism and make it even harder to lose weight. Researchers in Japan compared 6 and 7 year old children who slept nine to 10 hours a night to children who got one or two hours less sleep each night. Those who slept less were almost twice as likely to be overweight.

Read more: http://www.livestrong.com/article/277627

Chapter Five

Overcoming Weight Loss Plateaus

During your weight loss journey, there may be times where you experience weight loss plateaus. Almost everyone reaches a weight loss plateau at some point in their fitness lives. Before we review some techniques to break a weight loss plateau, we must understand why it happens.

Your body desires to be in a state of homeostasis, it does not like change. When change occurs it has to work harder. The human body works hard to keep energy intake and output in balance. In essence, your body does *not* like to lose anything including weight.

After your initial weight loss, your progress will slow down and eventually stop even though your exercise and food intake is consistent. This means that in order to lose more weight, you need to increase activity or decrease the calories you eat. Using the same approach that worked initially will maintain your weight loss, but it won't lead to more weight loss. Let's review some techniques that may assist with breaking your plateau.

Breaking Plateaus Technique 1

Trick your body. Switch up your workout routine. If you're using the treadmill or an exercise bike, do something different. If you are constantly doing the same exercises over and over again; your body knows what to expect. It's called "specificity of training." If you work out at a gym, change your cardio routine by getting on a stair-climber, an elliptical, or a rowing machine. Try ten minutes of intense cardio work on a machine and then switch and repeat. Mix up your workout so it's not a routine.

Breaking Plateaus Technique 2

Change your diet for a day or two. Take a day and alter your diet. Eat a steak if you haven't had one in months. You may even consider having a slice of cake or some homemade cookies. This drastic change in food intake will cause a shock to the digestive processes. A lot of times this is all the body needs to adjust the metabolism and get it back into overdrive.

If you decide to use this technique, please do so with caution. Depending on your weight loss diet, it may cause your body to reject refined sugars and fats. Don't utilize this technique as an excuse to go on a binge and eat everything you possibly can. You are only looking to shock your system, not send it into a weight loss disaster.

Breaking Plateaus Technique 3

Zigzag Your Calories. Although you may be staying on course with your weight loss plan, however by consuming the same amount of calories every day, your body weight can actually hit a plateau and remain at a standstill. If your caloric intake is 1300 calories per day, then your body simply adapts to take amount and stops losing weight.

To keep your body working hard at shedding excess pounds, vary the amount of calories you take in. Consume 1,300 calories one day; then reduce to 1,100 calories the next day; and 1,000 calories the following day. Keep this pattern going and your body will have to exert more energy to make adjustments, which can trigger greater weight loss results.

Breaking Plateaus Technique 4

Reduce your carbohydrates. By lowering your carb intake down to a ketogenic level it forces your body into a fat burning mode. This works best if you aren't already on a low carb diet (less than 100g per day).

Try lowering your carb intake to 20-40g per day for about 2 weeks whenever you hit a plateau. This is said to be the most difficult of all of the techniques, but also the most shocking to your body.

Chapter Six

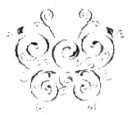

The Plan That Worked For Me

Without a plan, it's impossible to reach your goal. You must devise or choose a plan to follow in order to lose weight. It just won't haphazardly happen by chance. You must have a plan and stick to it.

My plan included cutting my caloric intake down to 700-800 calories per day. This is considered a very low calorie diet. If you decrease your calorie intake to this range, it is important that you obtain your doctor's consent. Obtain the proper nutrients on this type of diet is very important. I made certain that I took vitamins and ate the proper foods to keep me nourished.

Taking in so few calories forced me to make the right food choices in order to get the most out of my meals. I had to decide what I was going to eat and what I was absolutely going to refrain from eating.

My Food Choices

PROTEIN

- Low Carb Protein Shakes
- Organic Chicken
- All Fresh or Wild Caught Fish
- Tuna (packed in water)
- Turkey
- Low-Fat cottage cheese
- Low-Fat yogurt
- Eggs (egg whites are lower in fat)
- Fat-free or low-fat cheese (in moderation)

FRUITS

- Apples
- Grapes
- Blackberries
- Blueberries
- Cherries

- Strawberries
- Cantaloupe

SALAD

- Romaine Lettuce
- Onions
- Mushrooms
- Green Peppers
- Tomatoes
- Low-Fat Salad Dressing
- Virgin Olive Oil and Fresh Garlic can be used as dressing

THERMIC VEGETABLES

- Asparagus
- Bean Sprouts
- Broccoli
- Cabbage
- Cauliflower
- Celery
- Eggplant

- Green Beans
- Greens (without smoked turkey)
- Mushrooms
- Okra
- Onions
- Snow Peas
- Spinach (sautéed in olive oil is the best)
- Squash (spaghetti squash is a nice substitute for pasta)

BREADS AND GRAINS

- Brown Rice (1 cup)
- Low Calories Light Wheat or Whole Grain Bread (35-40 Calories Per Slice)
- Oatmeal

  (I love McDonald's Oatmeal without brown sugar.)

SNACKS

- 8-10 Almonds or Walnuts
- 3 Tablespoons of Trail mix
- 90 Calorie Special K Bars
- ½ cup of low-fat cottage cheese

- 1 cup of no sugar added peaches
- 1 cup of no sugar added mandarin oranges
- 1 cup of popcorn (no butter or oil) periodically
- Sugar free gelatin

FOOD FLAVORINGS, SEASONINGS AND SPICES

- Fresh Lemon/Lime Juice
- Olive Oil (1 to 2 tablespoons per serving)
- Garlic Powder
- Onion Powder
- Curry Powder
- Mrs. Dash
- Any light or fat-free salad dressing
- Salsa
- Sea Salt
- Black or White Pepper
- Truvia or Stevia Sugar Substitute
- Black or White Pepper
- Pam Cooking Spray
- Sodium-free is best

DESSERTS

- 90 Calorie Fiber One Brownie
- 100 Calorie Right Bites
- Fat-free or Lite Cool Whip (2 tablespoons)
- Sugar-free Popsicles

Foods I Chose To Avoid

- All Fried Foods
- All Potatoes
- Potato Chips
- White Flour
- White Bread
- Noodles and Pasta
- Pork
- Beef
- High Sodium Foods
- High Fat Foods
- Foods High In Sugar
- Candy, Cakes, Cookies, Pies and Ice Cream
- Foods High In Carbohydrates

Establish An Eating Curfew

I also established a rule which is what I call an eating curfew. I committed to no eating after 6pm. Adhering to this guideline required lots of self-discipline and a great amount of willpower. Many days, I would have to speak to my mind and tell it that it was not hungry then subject my flesh to my rule. ABSOLUTELY no eating after 6pm. I had come to the conclusion that I would not die by not eating pass my curfew and that I would eat the next day. After much practice, this became a habit and became easier to live by.

During times of temptation, if I got hungry and decided to eat, I made certain I ate extremely light and refused to eat beyond 8pm. I would have a piece of fruit, a cup of vegetables, or a small amount of almonds or trail mix to curb my appetite coupled with a glass of distilled water.

Drink Choices

By choice, I decided to drink nothing but water.

Water by far is the healthiest beverage that exists. Research does suggest that drinking plenty of water may help you lose weight. Dr. Brenda Davy, associate professor of human nutrition, foods and exercise at Virginia Tech, presented findings at an obesity conference which showed that people who drank two glasses of water 20 to 30 minutes before every meal lost weight more quickly initially and lost significantly more weight than those who didn't.

In another study by Davy, published in the Journal of the American Dietetic Association, she discovered that people who drank water before meals ate an average of 75 fewer calories at that meal. This may not seem very small and insignificant, but if you ate 75 fewer calories at lunch and dinner for the next year, you could lose about 14 ½ pounds. Water is very important and extremely important if you desire to lose weight. You must remain well hydrated. Being even 1% dehydrated can cause a significant drop in metabolism, which can also interfere with weight loss.

Water is also the best beauty treatment. You've heard this since high school, and it's true. Water will do wonders for your looks! It flushes out impurities in your skin, leaving you with a clear, glowing complexion. It also makes your skin look younger. Skin that is becoming saggy, either due to aging or weight loss, plumps up very nicely when the skin cells are hydrated.

I drink at least 1 gallon of water per day. You will go to the restroom quite frequently so be prepared. You are being flushed and cleansed. If you get tired of the taste, I would suggest adding fresh lemons, limes, sliced oranges, strawberries or even cucumber for extra flavor.

Again, drinking water only was my personal choice; however there are many others that drink diet sodas, sugar free flavored drinks, teas and coffees and still have managed to lose weight. It's a matter of preference. If you decide to drink a sugar-free beverage, limit to no more than 3 cans per day.

Chapter Seven

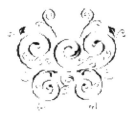

Daily Menus & Meal Plans

Here are some menus or meal plans that I used that may be helpful and enjoyable to you.

Day 1 Menu

Breakfast	Chocolate Protein Shake w/ 1 tablespoon of peanut butter
Lunch	5 ounces of baked chicken 1 cup of organic green beans
Snack	1 red apple

(Slice the apple, sprinkle cinnamon on it and heat it in the microwave)

Dinner	½ to 1 cup of low-fat cottage cheese 1 cup of no sugar added peaches
Dessert	1 sugar-free gelatin 1 tablespoon of Cool Whip Lite

Breakfast   1 cup of Oatmeal with cinnamon

Lunch   5 ounces of broiled salmon
                                   1 cup of steamed broccoli

Snack   1 cup of green grapes

Dinner   5 ounces of organic chicken breast
                              1 cup of steam cauliflower

Dessert   90 Calorie Bite Right
                             2 tablespoons of Cool Whip Lite

Breakfast

½ to 1 cup of low-fat cottage cheese
1 cup of no sugar added peaches

Lunch

4 ounces of tuna with fat-free
mayonnaise and chopped onions
2 large leaves of romaine lettuce
1 slice of low calorie wheat bread toasted

Snack

1 cup of strawberries

Dinner

Chef salad
2 cups of romaine lettuce
red onions
cucumber
4 ounces of sliced turkey breast
low-fat ranch dressing

(Fat-free or low-fat cheese is optional and should be used in moderation.)

Utilize the List of Foods That I Used To Create Your Customized Menus

Breakfast

_____

_____

Lunch

_____

_____

Snack

_____

_____

Dinner

_____

_____

Dessert

_____

_____

61

Utilize the List of Foods That I Used To Create Your Customized Menus

Breakfast   _____

_____

Lunch   _____

_____

Snack   _____

_____

Dinner   _____

_____

Dessert   _____

_____

Breakfast _____

_____

Lunch _____

_____

Snack _____

_____

Dinner _____

_____

Dessert _____

_____

Utilize the List of Foods That I Used To Create Your Customized Menus

Breakfast

_____

_____

Lunch

_____

_____

Snack

_____

_____

Dinner

_____

_____

Dessert

_____

_____

Utilize the List of Foods That I Used To Create Your Customized Menus

Breakfast   _____

                             _____

Lunch   _____

                             _____

Snack   _____

                             _____

Dinner   _____

                             _____

Dessert   _____

                             _____

Utilize the List of Foods That I Used To Create Your Customized Menus

Breakfast _____

_____

Lunch _____

_____

Snack _____

_____

Dinner _____

_____

Dessert _____

_____

Breakfast

_____

_____

Lunch

_____

_____

Snack

_____

_____

Dinner

_____

_____

Dessert

_____

_____

Utilize the List of Foods That I Used To Create Your Customized Menus

Breakfast

_____

_____

Lunch

_____

_____

Snack

_____

_____

Dinner

_____

_____

Dessert

_____

_____

Breakfast   _____

_____

Lunch   _____

_____

Snack   _____

_____

Dinner   _____

_____

Dessert   _____

_____

Utilize the List of Foods That I Used To Create Your Customized Menus

Breakfast

_____

_____

Lunch

_____

_____

Snack

_____

_____

Dinner

_____

_____

Dessert

_____

_____

Utilize the List of Foods That I Used To Create Your Customized Menus

Breakfast

_____

_____

Lunch

_____

_____

Snack

_____

_____

Dinner

_____

_____

Dessert

_____

_____

Breakfast   _____

                             _____

Lunch   _____

                             _____

Snack   _____

                             _____

Dinner   _____

                             _____

Dessert   _____

                             _____

Chapter Eight

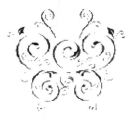

Encourage Yourself

Don't be so hard on yourself and enjoy the journey. We are typically our biggest enemy and our greatest critic. Instead of constantly criticizing yourself with negative, degrading comments, encourage yourself. Remain positive and jovial about who you are and what you shall become. Speak life into your success and consistently keep a winning mindset. Remain optimist at all times. "The optimist lives on the peninsula of infinite possibilities; the pessimist is stranded on the island of perpetual indecision." – W. Ward. If you endeavor to be optimist at all times then the possibilities of achievement are endless. Nothing will be impossible to you if you believe. You will receive your desired results and achieve your planned success.

Motivate yourself by looking at old pictures that show how large or overweight you were. Take pictures regularly, several times per week and use them to compare where you are in relation to the size you use to be. By looking at the evolving forever changing you, it will inspire you never to return again to the old, outdated, overweight, obese you. Share your pictures with others that support your process and allow them to join in on the celebrating your weight loss accomplishments.

Read inspiration scriptures and quotes daily. These will help your mind to become renewed. If your mind is not renewed, as you lose weight, mentally you will still think that you're fat. You will ultimately become discouraged and minimize your success. Nothing will ever be enough as long as you have your old mentality and think the way you use to think. You need a new mind with your new body!

Here are some scriptures and quotes that will help encourage you and keep you on course.

Inspirational Scriptures

3 John 1:2 - Beloved, I wish above all things that thou mayest prosper and be in health, even as thy soul prospereth.

Hebrews 12:1 - Wherefore seeing we also are compassed about with so great a cloud of witnesses, let us lay aside every weight, and the sin which doth so easily beset us, and let us run with patience the race that is set before us.

Philippians 4:13 - I can do all things through Christ which strengtheneth me.

1 John 4:4 - Ye are of God, little children, and have overcome them: because greater is he that is in you, than he that is in the world.

Romans 8:37 - Nay, in all things we are more than conquerors through him that loved us.

2 Corinthians 2:14 - Now thanks be unto God, which always causeth us to triumph in Christ, and maketh manifest the savour of his knowledge by us in every place.

Romans 12:1,2 - I beseech you therefore, brethren, by the mercies of God, that ye present your bodies a living sacrifice, holy, acceptable unto God, which is your reasonable service. And be not conformed to this world: but be ye transformed by the renewing of your mind, that ye may prove what is that good, and acceptable, and perfect, will of God.

Hebrews 12:11 (Amplified Bible) - For the time being no discipline brings joy, but seems grievous and painful; but afterwards it yields a peaceable fruit of righteousness to those who have been trained by it [a harvest of fruit which consists in righteousness--in conformity to God's will in purpose, thought, and action, resulting in right living and right standing with God].

Psalm 107:9 - For he satisfieth the longing soul, and filleth the hungry soul with goodness.

Isaiah 40:31 - But they that wait upon the LORD shall renew their strength; they shall mount up with wings as eagles; they shall run, and not be weary; and they shall walk, and not faint.

Romans 14:17 - For the kingdom of God is not meat and drink; but righteousness, and peace, and joy in the Holy Ghost.

2 Corinthians 5:17 - Therefore if any man be in Christ, he is a new creature: old things are passed away; behold, all things are become new.

Philippians 1:6 - Being confident of this very thing, that he which hath begun a good work in you will perform it until the day of Jesus Christ.

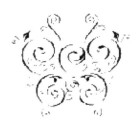

Motivational Quotes

Take care of your body. It's the only place you have to live. - Jim Rohn

The rest of the world lives to eat, while I eat to live. - Socrates

Living a healthy lifestyle will only deprive you of poor health, lethargy, and fat. - Jill Johnson

One way to get thin is to re-establish a purpose in life. - Cyril Connolly

Rule your mind or it will rule you. – Horace

The first and the best victory is to conquer self. - Plato

Gluttony is an emotional escape, a sign something is eating us. - Peter De Vries

The time for action is now. It's never too late to do something. - Carl Sandburg

Instead of giving myself reasons why I can't, I give myself reasons why I can. - Unknown Author

Never, never, never, never give up. - Winston Churchill

You don't drown by falling in the water. You drown by staying there. – Unknown Author

Our greatest weakness lies in giving up. The most certain way to succeed is always to try just one more time. - Thomas A. Edison

Motivation is what gets you started. Habit is what keeps you going. - Jim Ryun

The difference between try and triumph is just a little umph! - Marvin Phillips

Your goals, minus your doubts, equal your reality.
- Ralph Marston

*The tragedy in life doesn't lie in not reaching your goal.
The tragedy lies in having no goal to reach.*
- Benjamin Mays

*Our greatest glory is not in never falling, but in rising
every time we fall.* - Confucius

*The world of achievement has always belonged to the
optimist.* - Harold Wilkins

*No one can make you feel inferior without your
permission.* - Eleanor Roosevelt

*No matter who you are, no matter what you do, you
absolutely, positively do have the power to change.*
- Bill Phillips

The future depends on what we do in the present.
- Mahatma Gandhi Eleanor

Chapter Nine

I Did It, So Can You

My Redefined Campaign has been such a blessing. I am walking in victory in so many areas of my life. I've conquered struggles that have persisted for years. I finally got the victory over obesity and poor health. Amazingly, I've lost 70 pounds and went down 5 sizes. What an awesome accomplishment. I was able to achieve these results in only 4 1/2 months.

In addition, sugar diabetes has been defeated. I don't take any medicine and my sugar is perfectly normal. My glucose levels range between 80-90 and never exceed 100 even after eating a meal. I feel better, I look great and I did just what I said. I am Redefined. I am comfortable with the skin that I'm in. I have more strength and stamina than I have had in over 15 years.

I no longer shop in the plus size store or visit the women's size departments. I am not limited to a certain selection of apparel. My new size affords me the opportunity to choose from a wide range of hot, sexy, sensual clothing that I only dreamed of one day wearing. My dream has become my reality.

You can do anything you put your mind to. If you stick with your process, then progress will stick with you. Going completely through your process, stimulates favorable progress. Don't give up! Even when it looks like it's not working, stay true to your commitment. Many days you will lose inches rather than pounds, but in the end it all adds up.

Enjoy your weight loss journey. Remain focused and keep your eyes on the road to victory. If you don't, you will wreck and this will become another crash diet that ended in utter disappointment. Keep looking ahead into your future. Make a conscious decision that you will never return to your past again. Forget everything that's behind you. No other previous diet attempt matters at this point. The only thing that is imperative is what you are doing today in order to become a better you tomorrow!

Your new regiments should not only last for a moment but hold onto them through your lifetime. Eat right and exercise all the days of your life. With long life, God desires to satisfy you. Enjoy your life to the fullest! Don't take it for granted by reverting back to poor eating ethics and lack of exercise. You are responsible for protecting the Redefined You. Guard your image and watch over your health. You are a precious gift and must be treated as such by others and even yourself.

Refuse to abuse your body by eating foods that are not healthy for you. Treat your body well and give it what it deserves. It will appreciate you as you make a commitment not to depreciate it! Your best days are ahead of you! You don't look like what you're getting ready to become. You look so much better in your future. You are only several days and a few months away from a brand new life! If you create a Redefined

You, you are sure to see a much finer you. You have what it takes to get the job done. YOU CAN DO IT!

My Weight Loss Success!

70 pounds gone in only 4 ½ months!

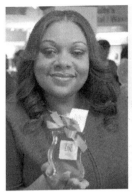 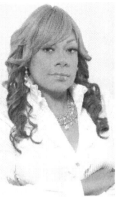

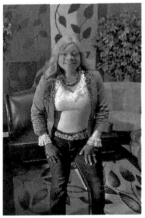

Before and After Pictures

Healthier

Happier

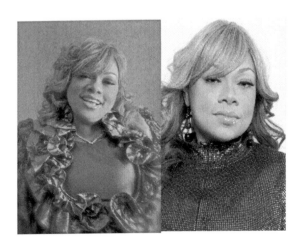

Sexier

Lighter

Made in the USA
Charleston, SC
11 November 2012